VERBAL DYSPRAXIA
IN
CLINICAL PRACTICE

VERBAL DYSPRAXIA

IN

CLINICAL PRACTICE

Betty Hill
LACST

Senior Speech Pathologist
Royal Talbot Rehabilitation Hospital
Melbourne

Distributed in the United States by

UNIVERSITY PARK PRESS
233 East Redwood Street
Baltimore, Maryland 21202

First published
in Australia 1978

Pitman Publishing Pty Ltd
158 Bouverie Street
Carlton
Victoria 3053

© Betty Hill 1978

National Library of Australia
Cataloguing in Publication Data

Hill, Betty J.
    Verbal dyspraxia in clinical practice.

    ISBN 0 85896 623 9

    1. Articulation disorders.
    2. Speech therapy. I. Title.

616.8552

Associated companies

Pitman Publishing Ltd
London

Copp Clark Ltd
Toronto

Fearon • Pitman Publishers Inc
Belmont, California

Pitman Publishing New Zealand Ltd
Wellington

Designed by Peter Yates
Cover design by Michael Payne
Illustrations by John Salter

Text set in 10/11pt Baskerville
by Modgraphic Pty Ltd, Bowden, SA

Printed and bound by
The Dominion Press, North Blackburn,
Victoria

PREFACE

This book is presented in response to the many questions posed by students and newly graduated therapists when faced with the task of producing an ongoing programme to restore articulation patterns in cases of acquired verbal dyspraxia. It is proposed that the book be used as a starting point from which the reader may develop and enlarge his or her own techniques.

On undertaking this ten-year study into the remedial and irremedial aspects of verbal dyspraxia, I hypothesised that only under certain conditions could such information be obtained. These conditions were:

1 A minimum of one hundred dyspraxic patients were to be treated.
2 The staff–patient ratio in the clinic would always be maintained at a level which ensured that every presenting dyspraxic received the optimum in terms of hours of therapy according to his current need.
3 Verbal dyspraxics of long standing who had failed to regain any purposive speech, with or without therapy, would be accepted for treatment. In this way I hoped to judge the efficacy of remedial techniques versus spontaneous recovery.
4 All patients were to continue therapy while gains were noted and the follow-up period to extend to a minimum of two years.
5 Full documentation was to be kept and would include medical history, initial test, full daily case history, weekly summary of progress, monthly retest and annual follow-up report.

One fact to emerge from the investigation, above all others, was that in terms of organisation and volume of therapy, dyspraxia is the most demanding of syndromes. It would be unrealistic for the newly graduated therapist to expect instant expertise.

This work is therefore the product of some six thousand hours of exposure to the problems of the verbally dyspraxic. The clinical realities of dyspraxia are but hinted at in current textbooks. Hopefully, this small text will be the first bridge over the gap between theory and practice.

CONTENTS

CHAPTER ONE

- **Incidence**
- **Spread of types**
- **Test patterns**
- **Prognosis**

An examination of the files of the 150 patients most recently presenting with articulation or language loss due to lesions in cortical areas showed an incidence of one-third verbally dyspraxic; aetiology was mixed. The highest proportion (38) had acquired their dyspraxia following cardiovascular or cerebrovascular incident, ten had suffered cerebral trauma and two cases were post-neurosurgical following removal of meningioma.

Further examination of the files of the 100 dyspraxics treated over the ten-year period showed the following spread of type:

1 Dyspraxia accompanied by sensory or global aphasia—32 cases.
2 Predominantly afferent or kinaesthetic* dyspraxia—36 cases.
3 Predominantly efferent or kinetic** dyspraxia—20 cases.
4 Efferent–dynamic dyspraxia accompanied by adynamia or lack of spontaneity—12 cases.

*SENSORY/KINAESTHETIC/AFFERENT DYSPRAXIA occurs when there is a breakdown in the post-central or sensorimotor area just posterior to the motor area proper. It presents as a defect of movement in terms of position in space.
**KINETIC/EFFERENT DYSPRAXIA occurs when pre-motor areas directly anterior to the motor zone fail to code or pattern successive movements. Individual, simple movement is carried out successfully but single motor movements are not synthesised into a smooth, consecutive action. Kinetic dyspraxia is a defect of movement in terms of time.

1

Table 1.1

DYSPRAXIA ACCOMPANIED BY DYSPHASIA

SPEECH INITIAL ASSESSMENT

Code: Severe (Total loss)   Moderate (50%)   Mild (25%)   Nil

Name ....   Date ....

Visual Agnosia   Agnosia present in varying degrees. Poor visual memory

Articulation	Loss		Loss
Dysarthria	—	*Dyspraxia*	
		Afferent	Severe
Dysphonia	—	Efferent	Severe
		Dynamic	Variable

Auditory Reception		*Expression*	
Phonemic hearing	Severe	Nominative	Severe
Retention of verbal traces	Severe	Reflective	Severe
Words	Moderate	Reactive	Severe
Simple sentences	Moderate	Narrative	Severe
Complex sentences	Severe	Automatisms	Variable
Paragraphs	Severe		
Conversational speech	Moderate		

Reading for Comprehension			*Writing*	
	Reading often			
Words	confined to	Severe	Copying	Often nil
Sentences	recognition only.		To dictation	Severe
Paragraphs	Matches words to		Initiation	Severe
	pictures			

Arithmetic	
Computation	Moderate
Problems	Severe

Attention & Retention   Attention may be satisfactory. Often severe losses of trace retention in all modalities

Estimation of length of treatment required for functional recovery of losses (Based on ½ hr daily therapy)   Indefinite
Degree of functional recovery expected   Nil unless acoustic integrity can be re-established
Remarks

2

Table 1.2

PREDOMINANTLY AFFERENT OR KINAESTHETIC DYSPRAXIA

SPEECH INITIAL ASSESSMENT

Code: Severe (Total loss)   Moderate   Mild   Nil

Name .... Date ....

Visual Agnosia   Usually presents with slower than normal scanning.   Nil visual agnosia

Articulation	Loss		Loss
Dysarthria	—	*Dyspraxia*	
		Afferent	Severe
Dysphonia	—	Efferent	Mild
		Dynamic	Nil

Auditory Reception		*Expression*	
Phonemic hearing	Nil	Nominative	Mild
Retention of verbal traces	Mild	Reflective	Severe
Words	Nil	Reactive	Moderate
Simple sentences	Nil	Narrative	Severe
Complex sentences	Nil	Automatisms	Often
Paragraphs	Mild		intact
Conversational speech	Nil		

Reading for Comprehension		*Writing*	
Words	Nil	Copying	Nil
Sentences	Nil	To dictation	Severe
Paragraphs	Mild	Initiation	Severe

Arithmetic	
Computation	Nil
Problems	Mild

Attention & Retention   Usually satisfactory

Estimation of length of treatment required for functional recovery of losses (Based on ½ hr daily therapy)   6–18 months

Degree of functional recovery expected   Moderately good but needs volume therapy to relearn articulation patterns

Remarks

3

Table 1.3

PREDOMINANTLY EFFERENT OR KINETIC DYSPRAXIA

SPEECH INITIAL ASSESSMENT

Code: Severe (Total loss)   Moderate   Mild   Nil

Name ....   Date ....

Visual Agnosia   Nil agnosia but occasionally poorly organised visual scanning

Articulation	Loss			Loss
Dysarthria	—	Afferent	*Dyspraxia* Usually *t–k* substitutions	
Dysphonia	—	Efferent		Severe
		Dynamic		Mild

Auditory Reception		*Expression*	
Phonemic hearing	Nil	Nominative	Mild
Retention of verbal traces	Mild	Reflective	Moderate
Words	Nil	Reactive	Moderate
Simple sentences	Nil	Narrative	Severe
Complex sentences	Nil	Automatisms Sometimes	Nil
Paragraphs	Mild		
Conversational speech	Nil		

Reading for Comprehension			*Writing*	
Words	Always needs to articulate to comprehend written material	Nil	Copying	Nil
Sentences		Nil	To dictation Variable from	Moderate
Paragraphs		Severe	Initiation Mild upwards	Moderate

Arithmetic	
Computation	Mild
Problems	Moderate

Attention & Retention   A mild defect of attention usually noted

Estimation of length of treatment required for functional recovery of losses (Based on ½ hr daily therapy)   3–6 months

Degree of functional recovery expected   Moderately good provided no severe degree of adynamia is noted

Remarks

4

Table 1.4

EFFERENT DYSPRAXIA—ACCOMPANIED BY SEVERE ADYNAMIA

SPEECH INITIAL ASSESSMENT

Code:　　　　Severe (Total loss)　　　Moderate　　　Mild　　　Nil

Name ....　　Date ....

Visual Agnosia　　Nil agnosia but poor visual attention and retention

Articulation	Loss		Loss
Dysarthria	—	*Dyspraxia*	
		Afferent	Mild
Dysphonia	—	Efferent	Moderate
		Dynamic	Severe

Auditory Reception		*Expression*	
Phonemic hearing	Nil	Nominative	Severe
Retention of verbal traces	Moderate	Reflective	Mild
Words	Nil	Reactive　Sometimes	Nil
Simple sentences	Nil	Narrative	Severe
Complex sentences	Mild	Automatisms	Nil
Paragraphs	Moderate		
Conversational speech	Nil		

Reading for Comprehension		*Writing*	
Words	Nil	Copying	Nil
Sentences	Moderate	To dictation	Moderate
Paragraphs	Severe	Initiation	Severe .

Arithmetic	
Computation	Mild
Problems	Severe

Attention & Retention　　Attention poor—well below normal

Estimation of length of treatment required for functional recovery of losses (Based on ½ hr daily therapy)　　Indefinite

Degree of functional recovery expected　　Prognosis poor if unable to initiate and monitor own errors

Remarks　　Patient often cannot maintain selectivity of traces to obtain correct name for objects—hence the nominative loss. Impairment to predicative aspect of speech affects narrative ability. In severe cases the speech is distinctly echolalic

5

The age range of the above patients was well spread from the early twenties through to the late sixties. The majority of cases were in the thirty-to-fifty age group. Age was not a significant factor in determining either the severity of the dyspraxia or the prognosis for recovery.

The initial test patterns of the four types were stable over the 100 cases, the only variation being degree of loss. They demonstrate both syndrome and prognosis. (See Tables 1.1 to 1.4.)

The prognosis for the remediation of verbal dyspraxia would appear to depend, not on the initial severity of the oral apraxia, but rather on the degree of spread of lesion into other areas of language or frontal function. Only five of the thirty-two global dyspraxics regained more than a minimal return of purposive speech. This despite a minimum of six month's intensive therapy and often a further eighteen month's maintenance therapy. The case history outlined in Chapter Nine should dissuade the beginning therapist from embarking on such a course with other than cautious expectations.

The type 4 dyspraxic, with the spread of lesion in frontal or tempero-frontal areas, appears equally irremedial. This depends always on the degree of adynamia or aspontaneity present. Those few with the aspontaneity confined to the production of articulemes only, as illustrated in Chapter Seven, usually respond well to graded trigger techniques and are reasonably remedial.

The remaining cases of kinaesthetic and kinetic dyspraxia as noted in types 2 and 3 all regained purposive speech in degrees ranging from a nearly normal return to a moderate result. But this was not without considerable effort on the part of both patient and therapist.

CHAPTER TWO

- **Introductory treatment in cases of severe oral apraxia**
- **Stage 1—establishment of acoustic integrity**
- **Stage 2—presentation of the concept of visual clueing**
- **Speed of progress**
- **Re-appraisal at the end of the first month**
- **Recognition of irremedial forms of dyspraxia**

The severity and type of dyspraxia should be carefully assessed but not without first establishing the present degree of neurological stability. Any test administered within four weeks of the date of return to full consciousness is suspect. A re-test at the eight-week level will often give an entirely different picture. If the patient is showing a severe degree of perseveration, and if trace retention is severely lowered in all modalities, neurological instability is indicated. If there is any doubt the same test should be administered on three separate occasions. Should the results show gross variance the patient is neurologically unstable and not yet ready for intensive therapy.

STAGE 1

Once satisfied that the patient is neurologically stable the starting point must be the assessment of his strengths and the establishment of acoustic integrity. Unless the patient is able to discriminate phonemes clearly, isolate them, identify them and eventually link them to graphemes, he will lack the ability to cope with the many hours of self-practice necessary for restoration of articulation patterns. It is best to begin at the minimum pair level. Provided the patient does not have an attendant acoustic agnosia he quickly identifies most words at this low level. Only the sounds close in articulatory formation and the voiced and unvoiced equivalents may give trouble. For example *d* and *n*, *b* and *p*.

Material needed for this exercise is listed below.

1 A complete set of minimal pairs, with all close initial, medial and terminal sounds featured in single-syllable words accompanied by brightly coloured simple pictures. These should be graded in order of difficulty, according to the closeness of the articulation process. Ideally, they are presented on *Language master cards* so that difficult ones may be practised for reinforcement.

2 Sets of pictured words containing three, four, five and six objects beginning with varied initial consonants and stable terminals. Example: *mat–bat–hat* working up to *tea–key–bee–tree–knee–d*. With them the patient's ability to isolate sound from a wider choice of alternatives will be tested. They may also be used later to refine auditory trace retention.

3 Sets of pictures accompanied by the written word, illustrating common objects with widely varied phonetic structure but of strong ideational value. Example: *dog–man–apple–bed*. With these the limits of the patient's auditory trace retention may be assessed. In the first instance he is required to point to one object. It is extended to two, three and four in the correct order. Unless he can achieve three, correctly ordered, auditory trace retention is extremely fragile. Four is the optimum for progress to the next stage of treatment. Anything less will indicate a temporal lobe deficiency which will not auger well for the patient's eventual prognosis.

Once the patient is achieving well in the above tasks, he is ready to abandon the pictured word and work with graphemes. Sets of written minimal pairs are now produced, beginning with those which have a widely varied visual and auditory aspect, working through to harder to distinguish terminals and medial vowels. The therapist demonstrates in an exaggerated fashion: **w**ay . . . **s**ay, **w**e . . . **s**ee . . . and the patient watches the therapist's mouth to note the visual difference in the initial consonant. He is then tested and points to the initial consonant 'observed' in a set of two. He does not need to be able to read the whole word to cope with this. The initial consonant is the clue. Once this is achieved his auditory capacity is tested. He looks away and still identifies the word heard. He proceeds then to the more difficult, but carefully graded visual–auditory discrimination tasks.

The rationale for such an approach to the problem of severe apraxia is three-fold.

1 As the patient is only involved in a listening task and has only to point to the consonant 'seen and heard' his area of greatest deficit is in no way threatened. (At this stage the patient is not expected to articulate the words.) Unless there is a severe temporal lobe

8

involvement he achieves quite well at this task and settles down, feeling pleased with the fact that he can at least accomplish in one area. It must be remembered that anxiety and frustration are characteristic of the dyspraxic.

2   The visual and auditory aspects of speech are brought to the forefront of the patient's consciousness. Unless he has a hearing deficit and has been forced to lip-read he will never have considered the visual aspect of speech. The auditory aspect, ie the isolation of phonemes and their link to graphemes, was lost around the age of seven, when he ceased to sound out words and began to read them as visual ideograms.

3   The therapist is able to assess other areas of deficiency which may influence the eventual remediability of the particular dyspraxic. Does he have a problem with sound discrimination? Is his auditory trace retention well below normal? Is his attention span limited? Is he able to retain an instruction or does he, in a task of discriminating between a set of w . . . s words, forget the visual clue for w versus s? If he passes all these tests easily he is ready for the next stage which is visual clueing.

STAGE 2

A chart is produced in which all the consonant sounds are classified and illustrated (photographically or with line drawings).

With the *lips*	With the *tongue*	With the *breath*
m	*t* . . . **d**	*h* . . . **h**
p . . . *b*	*k* . . . **g**	
w	**l**	
	n	
	r	
With *breath + teeth*	*breath + lips + teeth*	*breath + tongue*
s . . . **z**	*sh* . . . **zh**	*th* . . . **th**
	ch . . . **j**	
	f . . . **v**	

The principle of some sounds being without voice, as opposed to their voiced equivalent, is carefully explained. Patients invariably react favourably to an overall view of the schemata—the mystery unfolds. They are given the chart to study overnight. The next day the patient is invited to watch a demonstration of the various sounds, seated beside the therapist in front of a mirror. The resort to the mirror as the arbiter of the visual check must be well established in the early days of treatment.

At this stage the patient is given to understand that some sounds will be very much harder to imitate than others but that he will always be

9

helped by the therapist, firstly with icing to increase his sensory feedback (thirty minutes before the session yields optimum results) and secondly with spatula and fingers. In this way, a close approximation of at least one sound each session is the aim. Firstly, it is established that he is able to recognise the sound both visually and auditorally. Let *m* be the sound. It is written on a card accompanied by a visual presentation and he raises his hand when he sees and hears it in a stream of *hay–lay– day–may* words. He then attempts the movement. If he fails with visual clueing, ideational clueing is then introduced. He is not permitted to perseverate on failed attempts. The next day his retention is checked. After a short revision the grapheme is written and he must find the appropriate oral movement without delay. If, after the careful instruction of the previous day, he has not retained, his remediability should be suspect. Severe defect of intermediate recall, ie medial or primary brain damage, is not remedial. A remedial patient will work through the various oral positions within the first month and *retain* them.

Some consonants will be less precisely rendered than others; at this stage the patient will not be capable of great precision due to defects of muscle tone which invariably accompany this lesion. He should be reassured that precision will come later. As yet, only the spatial component of articulation, ie the direction in which the patient moves his lips and tongue to obtain the various consonants, is being attempted.

The therapist must not be tempted to obtain a consonant and to work on it to the exclusion of others for several days. This way lies disaster in the treatment of 'early days' dyspraxia. It will become so ingrained that the patient will perseverate on it indefinitely; it will become intrusive. By lowering the threshold for those patterns which are easier for the patient to obtain the threshold is automatically raised for those most difficult. Reinforcement comes much later in the programme.

If the patient does not have a total oral apraxia and has retained some automatic speech patterns, it is best not to have him counting, saying the days of the week and so on, in the hope that it will lead to better things. During early experience with the syndrome, a cherished hope that those preserved patterns would be the means of obtaining purposive speech did not prove to be so. Automatic speech exists at a level far removed from that of initiated, purposive speech. The aim must always be the conscious control of speech mechanisms, not to raise the already dominant level of automatisms. Much later they may be useful to illustrate a difficult sound combination.

Students invariably ask, 'which sound will I tackle first?'. The aim is to tackle them simultaneously. In this way there will be awareness of the particular difficulties of individual patients. No two will be exactly the same. *Herein lies the skill of the true remedialist—the ability to recognise individual patterns.* If the patient's defect of muscle tone tends towards flaccidity, the consonants *t–d–k–g* will prove to be of particular difficulty while *s–ch–j* will also give trouble. If, on the other hand, the patient shows a tendency towards spastic tone, these sounds will be easily obtained but *l* and *sh* will cause endless problems. If the efferent element is strong, all diphthongs, triphthongs and any sounds which require a series of movement (*w–ch–j*) and all blends, will prove particularly trying. Of all oral movements, for some reason not entirely ascertained, *f–v* released on to blends have proved the most difficult. (Thirty case histories attest to this.)

At the end of the first four weeks of treatment is the time for re-appraisal. Has acoustic integrity been established or is the dyspraxic so burdened with temporal lobe deficiency that he is unable to identify the sounds he is attempting to articulate?

Is he able to comprehend the therapist's instructions? Later on, when blends are introduced, they are going to become, of necessity, rather sophisticated. Does he really understand only one word in six, using the guess-technique for the remainder?

Alternatively, has he a deficiency in anterior areas? Is his attention span and control so fragile he is unable to settle to the task of obtaining control of oral praxis through visual clueing? Or does he need a constant reminder to 'look in the mirror'? Does he perseverate wildly?

Experience has shown that unless a patient has established acoustic and auditory integrity and at least an attempt at all phonemes in isolation, within the first month of therapy, he is unlikely to be eventually remedial. At this stage the therapist must appraise the situation. There will be pressure from relatives and the referring medical specialist to produce a prognosis and a result. The therapist alone can assess the advisability of continuing treatment. Either the patient is progressing well with daily gains, however small, and an established rationale for further treatment or he is a patient of doubtful remediability. Should the patient be rested and re-tested in three months in the hope that he has made gains in spontaneous healing and neurological stability? Should the therapist yield to external pressures and continue treatment in the hope that a miracle may occur, or have the courage to state that there is no rationale for continued treatment of this patient, devoting time, instead, to those with an obvious prognosis of remediability?

The therapist must make the decision. If the 'supportive' role has been opted for, then by all means therapy may be continued. If the therapist aims to be a remedialist, a more scientific approach must be adopted. Restoration of articulation patterns to the oral dyspraxic is not an exercise for the 'supportive' therapist (who manages the patient on a once or twice-weekly sessional basis).

11

CHAPTER THREE

- **Afferent dyspraxia**
- **Initial acquisition of consonant positions**
- **Difficulties encountered when attempting to impose movement patterns on faulty muscle tone**
- **Inhibiting effect of habitual patterns**

Although current literature defines afferent or kinaesthetic dyspraxia as a defect of sensorimotor areas and implies it may exist symptomatically as a separate entity from defect of premotor zones, this only occurred in ten of the thirty-six cases treated. These showed solely afferent characteristics. The remainder exhibited a mixed syndrome with widely varied elements of sensory loss plus kinetic difficulties. Nevertheless, in all cases with a strongly afferent element the starting point must inevitably be the production of single consonants, and to this end we shall consider their initial acquisition. Although vowel sounds may be used for mouth shaping they are not stable in their relationship to graphemes so are not considered in the initial instance.

m　should not prove difficult. It is most visible and the humming of a song (the right temporal lobe is usually functional) will ensure an immediate entrée. If the efferent element is strong it will be a difficult sound from which to obtain release.

b　is best obtained from m. It is often easily triggered from *umber . . . bu . . . bu* or *amber . . . ber*. Otherwise a visual demonstration of puffed-out cheeks, firmly closed lips and a firm pinch to the nostrils will obtain the movement. This is tedious and ideational acquisition is preferable.

p　is normally obtained from a demonstration of quick, gentle attempts to extinguish a match. Initially, the steady breath of the w will be presented. An admonition to start from a closed mouth and 'do it quickly' will usually suffice.

w has been found one of the easiest to obtain, although a double movement, and is often used as a starting point. A mere shaping of the lips by the therapist, a steady blowing of a candle flame and a sharp release assisted by the therapist's tap under the patient's chin, will normally be successful

l is another sound assisted by the integrity of the right temporal lobe. It is often immediately obtained from *la–la–la* to a popular tune. If the tone is spastic *da–da–da* will present and this substitution will alert the therapist to the order of presentation of sounds.

t can be most difficult in cases of flaccid tone. The alternate *k* will always be in conflict with *t* in the early days. It can be experimented with in several ways:

- As a terminal, following *n* as in *aunty . . . tea . . .*
- With strong ideational assistance as in *water . . . tu . . .*
- If the tone is spastic, it is most easily obtained from the sibilant *s* as in *star . . . tar . . . tar.*
- Only occasionally may it be obtained from the automatism *. . . one–two . . . two . . . two.* It is usually extremely difficult for the patient to isolate it.
- If the patient has a strongly afferent or sensory element to his dyspraxia, icing and the admonition to bite the tip of his tongue until it hurts may be successful in increasing the sensory feedback to the point where he can 'feel where it is in space' and produce the required movement.

d usually gives less trouble. It is usually obtained as a terminal following *n* as in *under . . . du . . . du.* If the tone tends towards spasticity *. . . mazda . . . da . . . da . . .* may offer more success.

k will always be in competition with *t* as a substitution. It is best attempted as a terminal: *anchor . . . ku . . . ku . . .* working on to *car* or *hanky . . . key . . . key . . .* have proved most fruitful.

g is similarly most easily obtained from *anger . . . gu . . . gu* or *hunger . . . gu . . . gu.*

r is also best obtained in the terminal position in the first instance. The therapist supplies the initial part of a word terminating in the *er* sound, eg bett*er*, butt*er* and the sound is refined from this point on.

s being a sibilant requires a certain degree of co-ordination between articulatory position and breath stream. If the tone is spastic it will probably present no problem, if flaccid, attention to the necessary rigidity of the tongue will prove a challenge. The tongue will fail to maintain a fixed position and a most slushy *sh* will probably be the fruit of the first attempt. A detailed description of a controlled attempt at *s* follows:

14

1 Place the teeth edge to edge (check in the mirror).
2 Part the teeth slightly, place a straw at the central point.
3 Wet the patient's hand and admonish him to blow down the straw until he feels the breath-stream on his hand.

Control and patience are essential.

sh is a most difficult sound if the tone is spastic. Starting from the 'teeth edge to edge' position of the *s*, the lips will need to be pushed forward by the therapist and the patient requested to attempt *shoe*. The *oo* vowel is the most facilitating.

th-**th** although visible are usually most challenging sounds. The combination of tongue extrusion and breath control plus rapid withdrawal appears difficult in concept. Isolated practice of 'tongue darting' without breath may be needed, working up to the combination of both.

f-**v** have emerged as the most difficult position for the oral apraxic. Although most visible, and the teeth may be neatly arranged on the bottom lip with the admonition to blow onto the chin, the release of the bottom lip and the simultaneous realignment of the teeth will need much patient instruction. Attempts at ideational acquisition have proved similarly disappointing. Although the patient may count to four with ease he invariably fails to isolate the sound. Obviously a 'latter day' phoneme.

ch-**j** prove difficult, indeed impossible, in cases of flaccid tone in early acquisition. If the tone tends towards spasticity they are easily obtained from the concept of a sneeze . . . *ah* . . . *choo*. With flaccid tone and a strong efferent element they can be left as the last acquisition.

n should give little trouble in the initial position except in cases of extreme spasticity or flaccidity. In the former a *d* will be substituted and relaxation must be obtained. In the latter case, tongue resistance exercises with spatula may be needed before the necessary pressure is obtained to distinguish it from the more flaccid *l*. It is a sound which needs special attention later in the terminal position.

It is preferable to be content, in the initial stages of visual clueing, with *one* correct rendition of the consonant position sought. The patient will attempt, in his enthusiasm, a repetition of the sound *ad infinitum* unless controlled. This will invariably result in a deviation as he will suffer a rapid onset of fatigue and consequent disappointment following his initial success, unless the therapist prevents this.

Every patient varies in the degree of assistance he obtains from the different sources, for example:

Visual clueing	The use of preserved automatisms
Tactile clueing	Verbal description.
Ideational clueing	

No simple formula can be applied to pre-determine this. The skilled therapist will experiment, observe and adjust techniques accordingly. Flexibility must be the keynote.

Speed of acquisition is vital, hence the need for at least twice-daily sessions in the initial stages. Anxiety is usual in the dyspraxic and although the aid of the physician may be enlisted and the patient suitably sedated, no current drug will produce the magic of sounds and eventually words, correctly articulated. The desire to communicate is inate in man. The oral apraxic suffers the ultimate form of frustration. Words tumble in to his ideational areas: he *knows* what he wants to say, but the appropriate articulation patterns are not conveyed to his errant tongue. At least the dysarthric can usually attempt an approximation of the sound. He does not have to listen to himself producing the bizarre substitutions which are the bête-noir of the dyspraxic. The therapist's skills will alleviate the patient's distress.

The inhibiting effect of habituated or low-level patterns can prove a challenge in early stages of recovery. Because of their common usage the threshold for certain patterns is lower and these will intrude automatically and disturb the ability to produce other sound combinations at will. For example, the word *park* will take precedence over all attempts to articulate its alternate *carp*. Therefore all words presented in the initial stage of therapy should be carefully screened and the test 'degree of common usage' applied. In this way, many a battle between the more common, or habituated pattern, and the more exotic will be avoided. There is time later, when control is better established, to challenge the patient with the latter.

CHAPTER FOUR

- **Re-establishment of articulemes as part of word patterns**
- **Reinforcement without perseveration**
- **Classification and categorisation as an aid to reinforcement**
- **Raising the link between grapheme and articuleme to the level of consciousness**
- **Self-practice**

Immediately a reasonable number of consonant positions are obtained in isolation it is necessary to assess the patient's ability to release these on to vowel positions. The use of varied consonants released on to a stable vowel has been found preferable to a stable consonant released on to varied vowels. Perseveration on consonant positions comes out strongly in statistical terms of 48 to 2.

On large sheets of newsprint, in much larger than normal script (to facilitate visual input) are printed:

MAY	*WAY*	*LAY*	*BAY*	*PAY*	*DAY*
ME	*WE*	*LEE*	*BE*	*PEA*	*D*
MORE	*WAR*	*LAW*	*BORE*	*POOR*	*DOOR*

As each rhyming word appears on the page the patient repeats the word after the therapist.

If the ability to sustain the selectivity of traces is poor, a group of four will be the initial limit. Remedial patients will soon be moving through the whole range, blends excluded.

During his early attempts at articulation, the patient is kept in a totally structured situation. Once he has attempted a word and failed, his cortical tone will be immediately lowered by his reaction of self disgust and frustration. He is not permitted to continue further attempts until he has paused a moment and re-assessed the requirement. The over-all aim is conscious control of an automatic process. Any repeated attempts at a failed articulation pattern will always result in perseveration of the initial misplacement. The therapist must supply this control in the early stage of treatment. The more remedial patients will acquire the necessary self-discipline within a reasonable period of time. The irremedial will unfortunately never attain it.

The next step must be the patient's ability to read from the rhyming sheets aloud, so he may commence *self-practice*. He has established acoustic integrity at an earlier stage. He is now mastering the ability to link a grapheme to an oral position. He must practise it to facilitate it and pass quickly on to the next stage.

By beginning with his most facile consonants and continuing to spend no more than one-third of the session on improving the production of his more difficult ones, the following procedure has been found most facilitating in the re-establishment of articulemes as part of word patterns:

W ... T
Water is   *wet.*
Black and   *white.*
Can't you   *wait?*
A bushel of *wheat.*

W ... D
A log of   *wood.*
Six metres   *wide.*
I give you my *word.*
A thistle's a *weed.*

Initially the therapist reads the phrase aloud, then repeats it, inviting the patient to join in on the *final* word, when he feels able. Once he becomes able to do this the therapist quickly withdraws assistance and triggers by reading the initial words of the phrase only. No more than four to five initial–terminal combinations are tried before moving on, as over practising at this stage will produce perseveration on the patterns to the exclusion of all else.

If the patient is remedial he will quickly begin to supply the word, quite often as the therapist is still writing the cue:

d ... g
A barking ...

Once single units are becoming well established, the therapist begins to extend slightly:

b . . . t
A little . . .   *bit.*
Place your . . .   *bet.*
I feel a bit . . . *better.*
A pound of . . .   *butter.*

It is necessary to move *quickly* and dismiss as unimportant those patterns he is unable to obtain at this stage. Success must be the keynote. No amount of soothing chats and murmers of sympathy will assuage the patient's frustration. Only successful articulation of words will calm him with the promise of better things to come.

Once the patient becomes facile at this low level the sound patterns he has achieved are written in his practice book. In this way, three large exercise books may be filled with:

a   All initial consonants to all terminals, example: *t . . . p, t . . . b, t . . . t, t . . . d, t . . . m, t . . . n.*
b   All terminals to all initial consonants, example: *p . . . t, b . . . t, t . . . t, d . . . t, m . . . t, n . . . t.*
c   If necessary, all short and long vowels with a stable initial consonant presented always in the same sequence and with varied terminals.

The advantages of this approach have been found to be four-fold:
1   Ideational areas assist in the facilitation of the attainment of the motor pattern of the word.
2   By the classification and categorisation of the graphemic structure the patient receives reinforcement in the task of raising the link between articuleme and grapheme to the level of consciousness. As he searches for motor patterns he begins to recognise his need for a *p . . . t* pattern, as opposed to a *p . . . m* pattern. His re-learning techniques are structured as opposed to random.
3   Reading and spelling, two areas of language function which have invariably broken down due to the missing articulatory link, receive simultaneous remediation. Note that in many cases no extra instruction has been needed, both areas making a good return with the re-establishment of articulation.
4   As the sound pattern is only repeated in a unit of four, the patient is receiving reinforcement without the danger of habituation and perseveration.

The patient is now, hopefully, capable of self-practice. Some patients have been capable of three hours a day, so motivated are they in their quest for verbal expression.

Once this stage has been reached, enough control of articulatory processes has usually been obtained to permit the introduction of such useful phrases as:

19

Yes, I do.   *No, I don't.*
Yes, I can. *No, I can't.*
Yes, I will. *No, I won't.*

The patient's ability to respond to questions directed to him with correctly articulated phrases is a morale booster which stimulates him to further effort. The patient is assisted by the alternates presented on printed cards. He is told the exercise is one of 'control'. He must attend to the question, select the appropriate answer and articulate it correctly. The therapist ascertains the likes and dislikes of the patient and structures the questions so that the response may be checked. 'Do you like tripe?', has never failed to elicit a negative response up to date! No attempt, however, has been made to link this to the esoteric aura of statistical research! As his ability to articulate improves, the patient could be required to extend the length of the sentence. The question, 'Do you like dogs?', could be expected to elicit the response, 'Yes, I do like dogs'. This could be an expectation at the 12-week level. He is not yet ready for initiated speech, but he is able to take an articulation pattern from the therapist and exercise enough control to structure a correct reply.

CHAPTER FIVE

- **Blends**
- **Pre-positioning problems**
- **Pre-release problems**
- **Vowels, diphthongs, triphthongs**

Once the patient is successfully tackling simple, single-syllabled words and confidently reading aloud from the rhyming sheets, it is time to introduce consonant blends. Only occasionally, to the therapist's delight, will a patient quickly master them. Many hours of patient instruction and practice will normally be necessary in remediation of verbal dyspraxia.

The difficulties encountered will vary from patient to patient and will depend on:

the degree of the afferent element;
the degree of the efferent element;
the degree of defect of muscle tone.

The largely afferent dyspraxic will encounter problems with pre-positioning. In articulating the word *tree*, he will fail to position his tongue medially for the *t*, thus giving himself a vast distance to travel to the blended *r*. The result will be *turee*, which, experience shows, is never refined into the required *tree* without the therapist's intervention.,

If the efferent element is strong, the patient is unable to plan the time element of the operation. He may position correctly but is unable to release the initial consonant quickly enough and monitor its smooth transition to the following one. Without the therapist's assistance he is not capable of pre-planning. His initial attempts will be *t* . . . (complete break) . . . *ree*, delivering them as two completely separate elements instead of a smoothly flowing whole.

With flaccidity of tone, blends which require little positional change but maintenance of a degree of tension in the muscles maintained over both consonants, as in *star*, will be the problem. The patient will either deliver the *s* . . . long pause while he recovers . . . *tar*, or the initial *s* will be completely omitted. Those with spastic tone will usually deliver *sar*, being unable to release the initial tension of the *s* to enable the articulation of the *t*.

To detail completely individual problems encountered in difficult releases would have to be the subject of a definitive work. Only the principles involved can be discussed in a paragraph. Firstly, it should be stressed that it is neither possible, nor indeed desirable, to present blends released to all allophones in the first instance. The individual patient's ability to perform more demanding oral movement returns through *levels* of sophistication. These are not necessarily strictly related to developmental levels. There are further dimensions to be considered in restoration of an impaired process. Not the least of which is the facilitation offered by ideational areas and the fact that, as a thinking and highly motivated adult, once he has experienced and established the sensation of the movement in an 'easy to obtain' position, he is often able to work towards the more difficult task of his own accord. The wise therapist's demands are graded according to the patient's present level and only those easiest to obtain are written in the practice book. The remainder can often be mastered during the practice of polysyllabic words or can be gradually introduced as a special exercise at a later date. Polysyllables will be dealt with in the next chapter.

In almost all cases, refining from a terminal acquisition with strong ideational assistance will offer the most facilitation. When refining to an initial position the *following vowel must be the most facilitating in terms of minimal demand of both positional and tensional change.* (Keeping in mind 'positional' for the strongly kinaesthetic-impaired and 'tensional' for kinetic impairment and defects of tone.) Some examples follow:

L **blends**   These would be attempted first in those with flaccid tone, last in those with spastic tone.

tl–dl   occurring as they do in the terminal position only, make a suitable introduction. The positional change is minimal and good ideational assistance is obtained from *bottle* and *handle*. Only those with severely spastic tone will find the abrupt change in tension difficult.

pl–bl   are best attempted from the strongly ideational *apple*, working on to *happily* and eventually refining to *plea* and the strongly ideational *please*. *Able* is refined in a similar way to *ably–blee–bleed*. If the kinetic element is strong, acquisition to open vowels in the initial position will require special attention. The ideational concept of *lay* is well established. The *p* element of the word *play* is described as having a half time-value only. The word is written as *p***lay** and attention paid to the momentary aspect of the *p* as opposed to the stressed **lay**. Such a course requires patient instruction but invariably overcomes the problem. The same measures apply, of course, to the *bl* as in *loo/b***lue**.

cl–gl   are not introduced until the *k–g* are well established in all positions and the positional conflict with *t–d* well resolved. They are best obtained terminally in the strongly ideational *ankle–angle*. The movement of the palate will assist in the acquisition of the *k–g* sounds which are always in conflict with *t–d*, and the move is made later to the initial position with open vowels.

sl–zl   present a challenge to those with spastic tone. The radical change from the tension of the *s* to the relaxed *l* will make this one of the later acquisitions. In the terminal position *hassle–muzzle* will usually suffice. In the initial position it is not wise to complicate the problems by requiring the patient to cope with a further change of tone by presenting a closed vowel as in *sleep*. An open vowel is by far the best initial facilitator. The strongly ideational *low* may have the half time-value *s* pre-positioned and *s***low** obtained. It is then often possible to work on through the various open vowels to the more closed ones, always keeping in mind the added value of ideational assistance.

fl   can be the most difficult of all blends to the afferent dyspraxic. It is usually the last attempted. In the first instance it is introduced positionally in the terminal position in such words as *awful–careful*, well before it is considered as an initial acquisition. It may sometimes be gained initially by working on to *awfully–flee*, but in many instances requires a careful positioning of top teeth, not over the bottom lip as in the case of the non-blended *f*, but slightly inside. Much patience is usually required to obtain the *fl* release. Possibly the simultaneous release of lip movement to tongue movement plus the change from breath to voice is the sum total of the difficulties encountered. However, once a dyspraxic easily articulates the word *flower*, he is well on the way to recovery.

R **blends**   These are not usually attempted until the *r* itself is well established in all positions. Those with flaccid tone will find them more difficult than the *l* blends. Some of the more difficult are summarised below.

tr–dr   is the best starting point. Once the medial position of the *t* is explained they will give less trouble. Initially they are best obtained in the terminal position with *water–under*, working on to *watery–Audrey* and thereon to *tree–dream*. The open vowels are attempted later.

cr–gr are also introduced terminally with *anchor–anger*. *Hickory–angry* will hopefully be refined to *cree–gree* and on to *cream–green*. The open vowels are also a later aim.

fr–thr because of the distance travelled are well established positionally in *offer–other* before attempting any initial acquisition; *fr* is sometimes obtained ideationally in the word *carefree*. With *th* a medial stage may be needed before proceeding to the initial, eg *other–mother–dither–dithery–three*. Open vowels are a later aim.

pr–br are introduced in *upper–amber* and if initial position is not obtained from these, it may be necessary to resort to the half time-value *p* linked to a strongly ideational word, as in the acquisition of *pl–bl* above. Closed vowels are attempted first.

str–scr are obtained positionally in the first instance from *mister–mystery–stree–street* and *whisker–whiskery–scree–scream*. Ideational assistance is often needed for the more open vowels, eg 'Don't go a*stray–stray–straight*.

kw is also a terminal acquisition. *Baker* is easily obtained, as is *wick*. The two are juxtaposed *baker . . . wick* and eventually refined to *quick*. In this exercise the phonetic **kw** is always written in colour or some other distinctive way above the initial *qu* word being practised. It has a definite, facilitating value.

tw a half value *t* is placed in front of *when*; *t***wen** leads on to *t*wen . . . *ty*. The word *twelve* is one of the most difficult and left for a much later date.

S **blends** It would be tedious to list these in the same detail. Those with spastic tone may find them easy of acquisition. They would be last to be introduced if the tone is extremely flaccid.

The *st–sp* and *sk* (the *t* and *k* element should be separated in order of introduction to avoid the substitution of one for the other) are normally acquired with *hasty–stee–steam . . . whisper–spur–spree . . . whisker–skir–skirt*. Initial position and open vowels follow. The *sn–sm* and *sw* blends are then introduced in that order. Strongly ideational words are well established, *no . . .* half time-value *s . . . s***now** *. . . might . . .* half time-value *s . . . s***mite** *. . . wheat . . .* half time-value *s . . . s***weet**. The patient is often invited to check the movement only without the added complication of breath-stream and voice, using the mirror. Patience and control will bring success. As these are all visible blends the patient will gain from self-practice and usually master them quickly.

Vowels may offer little problem to some, and once consonants are mastered the sensory dyspraxic will succeed with vowels ideationally from practice with the rhyming sheets. If, however, a strongly efferent or pre-frontal element is present problems may occur. Diphthongs and triphthongs presenting, as they do, the necessity to smoothly travel from one rather indefinite, and unfortunately not visible, position to another, may cause endless difficulties for the efferent dyspraxic. Considerable explanation will be necessary before they are finally mastered. If a pre-frontal element is added to his problems it will be seen in the inability to maintain 'systems'. The patient will commence practice on the rhyming sheets and maintain a diphthong for the first three or four words. The pattern will break down and a substitute sound appear. If this deficiency persists for a long time, past the three-month period, the prognosis for eventual remediability is questionable. Although diphthongs and triphthongs may be broken down into their separate elements and patiently explained, their acquisition and re-establishment as a necessary part of speech patterns must remain one of the most challenging aspects of the therapist's art.

CHAPTER SIX

- Efferent dyspraxia
- The facilitation offered by ideational areas when attempting to overcome difficulties in pre-release
- The technique of a stable prefix released to varied terminals as an introduction to polysyllabic words
- The value of the phonetic aspect of words presented as an aid to the acquisition of difficult syllables
- Defects of stress and rhythm
- The phrase and its eglided aspect

Although the majority of presenting dyspraxics will exhibit some afferent aspect in the first instance, the efferent or kinetic element will loom as a further challenge once the single-syllabled word is mastered. Occasionally a purely efferent dyspraxic presents. His ability to cope with the positioning of isolate articulemes is good, in imitation. His problem is one of release to varied terminals, polysyllabic words and correctly articulated narrative speech. He is unable to pre-plan release, in terms of time, to allow a smooth transition from one element of an oral movement to the next. Unless one element, including voicing and de-voicing, can be released at the appropriate moment to allow the commencement of the following pattern, no consecutive flow of smooth movement is possible. Initially, this must be *planned for him* by introduction of *carefully graded tasks*, with *strong ideational assistance and ever-increasing demand.*

The rhyming sheets are a good starting point if the problems are severe. These may be graded from simple words containing short and long vowels to words containing blended initial or terminal sounds. Blends followed by diphthongs and triphthongs follow and the number of movements within the word is increased. Terminal *l* following *oi* as in *oil–boil–spoil* proves a particularly difficult one in many cases, as does *fuel–cruel.* In the initial stages the cue is supplied by the therapist who reads across the sheet with the patient repeating each word after it is

27

read. Individual problems are noted and the 'time' element explained. He is then persuaded to read them aloud without assistance. During this process the therapist is able to assess the patient's particular difficulties so that the remedial techniques may be graded. This allows the therapist to assess degree of control and any tendency towards perseveration. If the patient achieves well at this level, words with a stable initial sound and a varied terminal are introduced:

heap . . . hear . . . heal . . . health . . . heave . . . heat . . . heater . . . heating.

The patient usually copes quite well at this level and is beginning to overcome his fear of extended articulation.

Compound words represent one short step forward. Beginning with such simple words as *house . . . wife, butter . . . fly, water . . . fall, arm . . . chair*, the second half of the word is covered while the ideational aspect of the first half is discussed. In turn the first half is covered and the second part tried ideationally. The two halves are blended into a whole. Although the patient is, in fact, only coping with two separate elements rather than a whole unit, he feels he is on the way to longer words and begins to lose his fear of them.

Analysis–synthesis sheets are now introduced. Words of two syllables, gradually working on to three, are written across the page with the stable prefix in colour or with an upper case–lower case or with any other method of distinction:

| *be***come** | *be***low** | *be***long** | *be***ware** | *be***side** | *be***tween** |
| *re***pair** | *re***turn** | *re***mind** | *re***move** | *re***lay** | *re***lation** |

The second syllable should have good ideational value in its own right. The patient reads each word aloud as he proceeds across the page. Stable suffix words with a requirement of two, three and then four syllables are then mastered. By this time such a strong ideational element is unnecessary but the phonetic aspect of words may need to be written, in a distinctive manner, over the graphemic presentation:

eks   peck   tay   shun
ex   . . .   pec   . . .   ta   . . .   tion

This will often have an extremely facilitating effect.

Unfortunately, the link between phoneme and grapheme becomes quite fragile in the English language, once proceeding to polysyllabic and more sophisticated words. An amusing aspect of efferent dyspraxia is the strong assistance rendered by ideational areas when attempting blending of extremely difficult syllables. One patient was totally bewildered by the motor patterns of the word *Australia* but achieved instant success with the assistance of the following explanation: **Os**, as in bone, **trail** as in trail bike and **yu** as in 'I'll be seein' yu.' (Non-Australian readers will no doubt fail to appreciate the dialectal aspects of this explanation!) It is probably not necessary to resort to such radical methods in many instances but it is as well to keep their value in mind.

Although, by this time, the patient is coping with words of several syllables he is often presenting them as separate units with complete absence of stress and rhythm. The concept of correct stress and its importance to the listener when interpreting the actual meaning of a word is introduced with these comparisons:

He has a foreign *ac*cent.
You must ac*cent* the second half.

He was an early Australian *con*vict.
The judge will con*vict* you.

I don't approve of your *con*duct.
He will con*duct* the orchestra.

Lists of words which stress the first syllable, second syllable or third are then practised. The patient now has the added requirement of considering correct stress as well as correct articulation. If this proves difficult for him the stressed syllable is always now written in upper case or other distinctive manner, when presenting material in the practice book.

Although this will assist him to produce the actual word with the required stress and rhythm, the sentence is often still delivered with each word as a separate unit, rather in the manner of consecutive bullets fired from a rifle. The eglided phrase is then practised:

bread 'n' butter
up 'n' down
fish 'n' chips
a cup 'v' tea
a pound 'v' butter

Extraordinary as this may look in print, it is nevertheless effective in stressing the need for an altered time element. Further phrases are practised using 'contractions':

I'm . . . awake
I'm . . . afraid
I'm . . . amused

Considerable time may need to be spent on these. It is necessary to stress that the last sound of the contraction be held until a smooth release on to the following word is gained. The voice must not be shut off.

29

Vocalisation must continue through to the following word. An occasional dyspraxic will find the smooth transition from voiced to unvoiced sounds troublesome also, but this is unusual.

During the exercise of releasing contractions to a word and then to a slightly longer phrase the move is made from the controlling influence of the written word to the production of initiated speech. If the patient is unable to do this, the material discussed in the next chapter will be of interest. Perhaps, on the other hand, while not actually adynamic, he needs a further time in a structured situation. The first move could be to present him with the alphabet and take it in turns with him to move through the letters, using each one in turn to trigger the first word of the phrase following a contraction:

I'll ask her.
I'll be there.
I'll come and get it.
I'll do it.
I'll eat my dinner.
I'll go for a walk.
I'll have a rest.

As he works through the various contractions (*I'm, I'll, I'd, he's, she's*) the patient could be required to work towards slightly longer phrases. In addition to this a little time may be spent on the production of the simple sentence in all its forms. Action pictures may be presented and the therapist's question 'what is the woman doing?' triggers the response 'she is ironing'. These are graded up to longer requirements: 'She is sitting under a hair dryer and drinking a cup of tea'. Simple requests are practised and the patient responds to a hypothetical situation supplied by the therapist: 'The television is too loud—what would you say?', 'A cold breeze is blowing through the room and you are seated a long way from the window—what would you say?'. Statements given by the therapist could be required to be converted into questions and vice versa: 'It's raining' converted to 'is it raining?' as a starting point, working on to the more sophisticated 'I bought a new car last week', converted to 'did you buy a new car last week?'. He may be required to provide a suitable ending to a 'non-triggering' introductory phrase: 'My mother . . .', 'Last night . . .' and to reverse the process by supplying the beginning of the sentence when provided with the final phrase: '. . . at the weekend'.

If he requires any further assistance in developing spontaneous speech at sentence and narrative level he is adynamic or has a dysphasia accompanying his dyspraxia. The afferent–efferent dyspraxic will, if there are no further complications, begin to produce narrative speech spontaneously once articulation patterns are relearned. In most cases his written narrative will also slowly recover once the articulatory link is restored.

In ten cases, with initial test patterns of inability to write words past single-syllable level accompanying the dyspraxia, no direct work on spelling was given in an attempt to test this hypothesis. All recovered their written language to the stage of coping with a short letter to friends by the time articulation was restored, and were able to go on from there with self-practice to improve their written texts. Only those with accompanying dysphasia were unable to do this. They, in turn, needed many hours of patient instruction in written, as well as spoken, language.

CHAPTER SEVEN

- **Adynamia**
- **Dynamic dyspraxia**
- **Graded trigger techniques**

The degree of impairment to other areas of frontal function co-existing with a verbal dyspraxia must have a strong bearing on the eventual prognosis. If the patient exhibits severe aspontaneity and the test pattern presents with all areas of language function severely depressed, prognosis is undeniably poor. A lesser degree of adynamia may also be revealed in the later stages of treatment of the efferent dyspraxic, when, despite good restoration of articulation patterns, he is slow to regain spontaneous speech. He may answer questions readily enough and be prompted into speech, but rarely initiates more than 'low level' greetings to his fellow patients as he moves among them in the rehabilitation setting.

There was another small group of only 8% of dyspraxics treated over the ten-year period whose adynamia appeared restricted to the production of the articuleme and spoken language, rather than an inertia spread over all modalities. In the initial test auditory areas presented as intact; they were able to read for meaning at nearly normal speed and most were able to write both words and phrases in initiation and from dictation. They were not easily able to read aloud what they had written, however. Naming, reading aloud and reflected speech all contained the substitutions and release problems of the typical dyspraxic. In conversational situations they often made no attempt to initiate speech, confining themselves to 'yes', 'no', responses, accompanied occasionally by gesture. The vital difference exhibited by this group from all other dyspraxics assessed was their immediate response to an ideational trigger. Although many dyspraxics are assisted by it in the early days of their recovery, to this group it was pure magic. This key unlocked their lost articulation patterns. To illustrate further, in a simple exercise naming a series of simple pictured objects, the words would be mispronounced or even no articulation pattern found. The addition of the printed word and the therapist supplying the articulation model to be copied would bring little improvement. However, as soon as the word was led in with a trigger—a barking . . . *dog*, a T-bone . . . *steak*—correct articulation patterns would immediately be produced for all words, even polysyllabic ones.

To remediate these patients an entirely different treatment plan was required. By carefully grading trigger techniques from totally predicative to those providing less associative or ideational support, it was possible to proceed to a gradual withdrawal, with the patient eventually providing his own internal trigger process. The actual treatment process was reversed. The 'regular' dyspraxic requires a calm, controlled approach during treatment sessions, any excessive demand inevitably leading to loss of control and perseveration. The dynamic needed to be stimulated with large quantities of pre-prepared material, delivered in rapid succession and to be kept in an atmosphere of excitation, with the therapist's voice positive and slightly raised.

An abridged case history of one such patient follows, with samples of the material used. Similar material may be effective in overcoming latent inertia of those dyspraxics who fail to regain spontaneous speech despite restoration of articulation patterns.

AETIOLOGY

Subarachnoid haemorrhage. The angiogram revealed aneurysms on the left anterior cerebral and left middle cerebral arteries. Both aneurysms were successfully clipped.

SEX & AGE

Female 44.

DATE OF PRESENTATION

14/52 postoperative.

TEST PATTERN

Decoding	Reception for the spoken and written word was intact.
Encoding	There was severe oral impairment. The patient could write from dictation and initiate the written word.
Automatisms	These were intact.
Spontaneous speech	Nil.
Strength	She responded immediately to a trigger with correct articulation patterns.

RATE OF PROGRESS & MATERIAL USED

Week 1 The patient was naming fifty objects with a supplied ideational trigger.

Week 2 She was supplying her own internal trigger for simple naming.

Week 3 She was supplying the verb for:

The sun is . . .
The wind is . . .
The phone is . . .
The dog is . . .
The choir is . . .
The tap is . . .
The jug is . . .

The patient still needed a highly predicative level of trigger.

Week 4 The patient was working from the highly predicative to the less predicative:

Look at the sun. The sun is . . .
Feel the wind. The wind is . . .
Is that the phone? The phone is . . .
I have a knife and a knife is for . . .
Here is a pen and a pen is for . . .
Look at my hair, it needs . . .
Hand me the broom and I will begin . . .
She has just heard a joke and she is . . .

working on to the 'two-word requirement' of:

My dinner is in front of me and I am . . .
I have a glass of water and I am . . .
My hands are dirty so I must . . .
The steak is raw so I must . . .
This chair is in the wrong place so I am . . .

35

The lawn has grown too long so I am . . .
She is throwing the ball and I am . . .

working on to a 'three-word requirement' of:

We disagree on the subject so we are . . .

Week 5   A simple statement was triggered in the following way:

The sun is shining! What is shining? What is the sun doing?
The dog is barking! What is barking? What is the dog doing?
The tap is dripping! What is dripping? What is the tap doing?
The jug is boiling! What is boiling? What is the jug doing?

working on to the less assistive:

This meat is tough! What is the meat like?
The windows are dirty! What is wrong with the windows?
I am very tired! How am I feeling now?
This work is difficult! What is this work like?
John is going home! What is John doing now?

At the end of the fifth week the patient began to initiate a simple statement.

Week 6   The patient was required to supply a phrase to end such statements as:

The milkman is . . .
The footballer is . . .
The mechanic is . . .
The butcher is . . .
The typist is . . .
The policeman is . . .

She was also required to supply a suitable subject for the following:

. . . is blowing.
. . . is servicing my car.
. . . is mending the water pipes.
. . . is counting the money.

Week 7   The patient continued to work with highly predicative adjectives and adverbs:

Look at that . . . rain.
Can you see the . . . stars?
They dashed into the . . . surf.
We sat before the . . . flames.
I'll cook some . . . eggs.

The children played . . . in the park.
The birds sing . . . in the morning.
Mary studied . . . for her examination.

During this period more sophisticated nouns were sought. Starting, of course, from the highly predicative and working towards those with less ideational assistance:

A fertile . . .
A correct . . .
A busy . . .
A lonely . . .
A rude . . .
A difficult . . .

There was now a choice. The patient had to suppress and select. Most of the remediated patients with this condition complain of the difficulty in selecting one appropriate word from a plethora of alternatives not of a lack of ideas. The patient is coping with the problem of *inhibition of alternatives*—always a problem with frontal impairment.

Week 8   To this end the patient was now given trigger with a less predicative aspect, and had to select from alternatives. Irrelevant ones had to be suppressed and the appropriate brought forward into the forefront of the consciousness. The following requirement was given:

Answer . . . (the alternatives are *letter, phone, question*). The patient must select.
Buy a . . . (the alternatives are endless).
Bring me a . . . (as above).
Make a . . .
Have a . . .
Look at the . . .
Pass the . . .

Week 9   The patient was ready for a phrase, starting of course with the more predicative and working towards those in which her own ideational areas had to supply the terminal.

Answer the phone . . .
Bring me a cardigan . . .
Wind your watch when . . .
Don't buy it unless . . .
Wait here until . . .
I won't be late unless . . .
He called the doctor when . . .
I'm crying because . . .

37

Week 10   The patient was ready for exercises in narrative. She was presented with a simple, controlled task. 'Tell me the steps you would take to make a cup of tea.' 'Tell me the steps you would take to change a tyre.' She had to sort and suppress. From a plethora of alternatives she had to supply the most appropriate phrase in its correct sequence in the overall plan.

Week 11   Only occasional misarticulations and hesitations were now noted in the patient's speech.

Week 12   The patient was discharged to job retraining.

Further therapy would be required and supplied at a higher level. The therapist's role, in this instance, was to 'pave the way'.

CHAPTER EIGHT

- Case history
- Restoration of articulation patterns in a case of oral apraxia

This case has been selected for presentation of oral apraxia in its most extreme form. No gains were spontaneous. Every articuleme, every word, every phrase was relearned. The patient spent over two thousand hours self-practising in the eighteen months he devoted to his quest for restoration of verbal communication. In doing so he has contributed to our knowledge of what is possible, in terms of remediation of oral apraxia.

AETIOLOGY

Left frontal meningioma. The patient presented with a history of severe headache over a period of one year and recent visual deterioration. Investigation revealed an extremely large left frontal meningioma lying adjacent to the motor speech area. This was removed leaving the patient with a profound oral apraxia.

SEX & AGE

Male 37.

DATE OF PRESENTATION

16/52 postoperative. Speech therapy was attempted postoperatively without success. The patient returned home to a country town and no

39

spontaneous gains were made. On presentation he was totally orally apraxic.

TEST PATTERN

- Strengths—Phonemic hearing was intact. He comprehended speech at sentence level. Attention and retention were good. There was no evidence of perseveration.
- Deficiencies—All areas of visual and language function showed some degree of impairment. Visually, he was slow to scan and unable to read for meaning past simple sentence level. He was also unable to form letters and write either to dictation or in initiation, other than at the level of kinetic ideograph (signature).

INITIAL PROGNOSIS

On the balance of deficiencies versus strengths his therapists were initially cautious. Despite experience in the field they had not learned to take into account 'sheer determination' and to devise a test for it. By the second day of therapy the patient's special qualities were becoming obvious. He had excellent retention and an incredible degree of control and patience, as he tried, firstly, gross oral movement and then articulemes by visual clueing.

TREATMENT PROGRAMME

First Month Day 1 Tests were carried out on the patient.

Day 2 His acoustic integrity was established.

Day 3 The principle of visual clueing was introduced.

Day 4 All consonants were attempted in isolation except *ch–j–th–f*.

Day 5 All consonants, except those above, were released onto vowels in rhyming sheets.

Day 6 Initial *p* words were released to all terminals, except those above, in groups of four with ideational assistance: *th* was introduced in isolation.

Day 7 Initial *b* was tried with all terminals; *f* was attempted in isolation, but was difficult.

Day 8 *p–b* were well established. *ch–j* were introduced in isolation. Automatic phrases: 'Yes, I do', 'No, I don't' were attempted, together with 'hello' and 'goodbye'. Articulation was not perfect but comprehensible.

Day 9   Initial *t* was introduced. This was difficult but the patient tried intelligently and always self-corrected. The usual problems were encountered when moving from tongue to lips in *t . . . p* words.

Day 10   Initial *d* to all terminals was introduced and this was easier for him. (It should have been introduced before *t.*)

Day 11   Initial *k* to all terminals was used.

Day 12   Initial *g* was tried. The patient was weak on *g . . . d* words. Reinforcement was needed.

Day 13   Initial *w* was introduced to all terminals. He was now reading simple learned phrases aloud.

End of First Month   The patient had worked through *n–l–f–th* plus the above sounds in the initial position released to simple terminals. He needed constant revision but was retaining well once mastered.

Programme   Two daily half-hour sessions of therapy. Two half-hour sessions of self-practice in front of a mirror, partly monitored from an adjoining room.

Second Month   Special difficulties were noted—initial *h*, terminal *g*, *m . . . n* words. Some ear training was needed when introducing *sh–ch* alternates. Terminal *st* was introduced. Initial *r* was well established and *r* blends commenced.

Third Month   The patient returned for further surgery (insertion of a plate). He was delighted by the surgeon's praise and surprise at his speech progress. (This was very helpful to the patient as, in fact, his articulation was still extremely laboured and somewhat painful to the ear.) By the end of the third month he had attempted all single terminals and was extending to two syllables and blended terminals.

Fourth Month   The terminal *f* and the terminal *th* both needed considerable reinforcement; *l* was mastered medially. *fr–fl* blends were given special attention. Attempts were made to initiate speech at the simple narrative level. The patient chose words carefully to avoid difficult releases and struggled on with his story. Speech was comprehensible but still painful to the ear.

Fifth Month   All blends were mastered. He was beginning on eglided phrases. He tended to break voice and found the task difficult. All terminals in the plural were introduced. *She'z* was giving the most trouble due to the abrupt change of tone; *thr* blends needed reinforcement and terminal *l* following triphthongs was a problem. The

41

patient also began reading words of two and three syllables from the analysis–synthesis sheets.

Sixth Month Longer periods were spent at home. A relative attended for training in assisting the patient with practice sessions and he worked with her for two hours each day on set work, mostly reinforcement of acquisitions during the latest period of therapy. Her assistance was invaluable.

He coped with polysyllabic words provided that phonetic structure was illustrated. Special work was given on the less phonetic terminals: *tious–tion–cient*. Speech was halting and obviously dyspraxic but no vocabulary loss was noted. He was definitely getting his meaning over at this stage, despite an occasional (always self-corrected) mis-articulation. He showed surprisingly little self-consciousness about his impaired speech and did not hesitate to initiate a conversation, even to strangers. He obviously had no adynamia.

Seventh Month Further refinement was needed on *f–v* in all positions; *few–futile–furious* were particularly hard for him. He could not obtain a smooth enough transition. Cardinal numbers, presenting as they do a terminal *th*, required special attention, particularly twelfth. He was now doing more than three hours a day of practice on polysyllabic words, phrases and sentences. Stress and intonation were not yet mastered.

Eighth Month The patient had now returned to the country with adequate material for structured practice over the next four months. He was to present two days a month for further work on more difficult patterns.

Twelfth Month The patient was reviewed. Speech was halting but correctly articulated. Further work was given on stress and egliding.

Eighteenth Month The patient was now re-employed. Contact was now mainly by correspondence. Written language had slowly returned, parallel with restoration of articulation. The letters in the file showed an interesting development from 'This is first letter I write you', at the sixth month of treatment to the fluent, well-spelled notes reaching the clinic at the eighteen-month stage.

PRESENT STATUS

Although re-employed by his previous semi-government body, the patient has had to accept a less demanding position than at his previous managerial level. He is well content with this for the moment but declares he will 'work on to better things'. Although his speech is moderately fluent it has a flatness of tone which has not yet been overcome. Consonants are always carefully pronounced but diphthongs and triphthongs are sometimes 'shaded'. One gains the impression that he has but recently learned the language but done so very, very thoroughly.

CHAPTER NINE

- Irremedial conditions
- Case history—Severe oral apraxia accompanied by acoustic mnestic dysphasia

The previous case history was offered to illustrate the formidable task, in terms of time, patient instruction and self-practice, encountered when attempting restoration of speech to the severely apraxic. It is as nothing compared with the problems which will present when apraxia is compounded by an attendant dysphasia. In many cases one will find the difficulties insuperable. The newly graduated therapist will be presented with many such cases and a request for remediation. Inevitably there will be some failure and then the question will be asked 'Was the failure mine—was there something further I could have done?'. The following case should be considered. One such patient was offered every possible assistance in terms of hours of therapy over a considerably extended period. She was young, alert and incredibly persevering. She had excellent family support. A brief resume of the difficulties encountered follows:

AETIOLOGY

A sudden onset of total aphasia–apraxia was due to emboli in the left middle cerebral artery, proved by carotid angiography. This occurred while parachute jumping, but investigation failed to reveal aetiology for the emboli. There was some accompanying (R) hemiparesis which made good recovery over six months.

45

SEX & AGE

Female 35.

DATE OF PRESENTATION

8/52 post incident.

TEST PATTERN

As in type 1 in Chapter 1.
* Strengths—The patient was quick to interpret gestures. She was alert, co-operative and determined.
* Deficiencies—No area of language function was intact.

TREATMENT PROCEDURE

Month 1 Exercises in visual and auditory discrimination were introduced. Some visual gains were made but despite instruction the patient did not discriminate even grossly varied sounds unless clued by oral movement. She was unable to retain the link between phoneme and oral movement. Auditory verbal comprehension was completely extinguished except for appropriate response to greeting. It was strongly suspected that the patient interpreted even these by intonation only. Some attempt was made to imitate gross oral movement.

Month 2 The patient could imitate some oral movements but was unable to link them to grapheme, or indeed to retain them in any way. Twice daily therapy and 30 minutes reinforcement on *Language master* in sound discrimination, linked to both pictured object and grapheme, were given.

Month 3 She was still grossly mnestic but could now imitate all consonants except *ch–j*; *s–sh* were weak but were attempted. *t–d* were in conflict with *k–g*. She was beginning to distinguish widely varied minimal pairs, and had mastered, in initial position, the following:

we . . . see
h . . . m
s . . . m
l . . . r
w . . . m

and was working with some success at the more difficult

t . . . k
g . . . d

s . . . sh
sh . . . ch
n . . . m
n . . . d
f . . . th

in sets of four with a long vowel following. The words were presented with attached pictorial illustration.

Month 4 The patient was becoming acoustically stable and identifying simple objects. She was still unable to retain grapheme shape and link to phoneme; she was grossly mnestic. There was no spontaneous speech other than 'yes' and 'no'. She was continuing to work on imitation of single sounds but was unable to release them to a following vowel.

Month 5 Finally, the patient had established acoustic integrity. She discriminated most sounds, terminal *t–p* and initial *sh–ch* were still tentative as was *n–d* and *n–m*. She was beginning to link phoneme to grapheme and to retain. She now had a unit of three in terms of auditory trace retention. One hundred hours of therapy and progress was only thus far!

Month 6 The patient was understanding conversational speech now at a very simple sentence level. She could not cope with extended narrative or command. She indicated that she was not yet neurologically stable. There was word perseveration and she was unable to dismiss the words from her consciousness so that she could attend to the following ones in a narrative. There was still no return of any automatic or spontaneous speech. Nothing was able to be triggered from ideational areas. She was determined to persevere.

Month 7 At long last the patient was able to cope with visual clueing, attaching phoneme to grapheme and reading simple words from the rhyming sheets. She was unable to form letters but structured simple words from dictation with alphabet cards.

Month 8 She was releasing all initial consonants on to all vowels in the rhyming sheets. Blends were started. There was still need for a totally structured situation to produce any articulation patterns and there was no return of speech outside the clinic. Comprehension was much improved, however. The patient was attractive and vivacious and did so well with mime. She was very popular with fellow patients.

Month 9 She was now coping with all initial sounds to all terminals in the structured ideational situation. *s* blends were causing problems but she was tackling them patiently. Despite the fact that she was now

47

regaining articulation patterns she was reluctant to initiate speech. She aimed always for perfection in articulation before she would attempt to use words to outsiders.

Month 12 The patient returned home. Many hundreds of hours of therapy had been given and she was only able to communicate in words and very simple sentences. Further management would be outpatient therapy with a relative continuing to assist her with practice.

Month 24 She was now able to telephone and hold a brief conversation. Her husband said that she thought out what news she wished to convey, wrote it down and practised articulating it for an hour or so before she attempted the telephone call.

Month 36 The patient had returned to work and coped quite well. She communicated at a limited level but was usually able to 'get her meaning over' provided that she was given time to structure her response, in a conversational situation.

Conclusion Severe dysphasia–dyspraxia is not readily remedial. Perhaps with a young, totally determined patient some limited degree of communication may be achieved under ideal conditions and with many hundreds of hours of therapy over an extended period. Unfortunately, in the large majority of cases, prognosis is extremely poor.

CHAPTER TEN

- **Conclusion**
- **Some aspects of patient management**

The inclusion of case histories of such extreme forms of apraxia should not discourage the beginning therapist. Apraxia occurs in all degrees, from the mild which shows excellent spontaneous recovery with minimal therapeutic intervention, to the severe and irremedial. It must be repeated that initial test patterns which indicate a severe spread into other areas of language function or severe frontal involvement do not promise well in terms of eventual prognosis.

Unless a patient is severely frontally impaired, motivation will never be a problem. He will pursue his lost articulation patterns to the point of exhaustion unless well controlled and will always demand more and more therapy. Although two sessions each day would be the minimum for speed of progress in early days, the patient would present for five if given a chance. Once he regains the ability to link phoneme to grapheme and commence self-practice (he is not at the beginning of remediability until this stage is reached) this too must be controlled and confined initially to short periods. Later, when he is better able to judge approaching fatigue, he may be allowed to extend the periods. He is a demanding patient, both of the therapist and himself.

One unexpected finding to emerge from the long-term study was the response to remedial techniques shown by *long-standing dyspraxics* who had failed to regain any spontaneous speech, usually after the initial six months or so offered in hospital clinics, and had been returned home

49

without further therapy for periods ranging from two to six years. Perhaps treatment procedures should be reassessed. At the moment it is usual to give the most therapeutic assistance in the early days of recovery. This is when cortical tone is often at its lowest and the ability to cope with trace retention is not yet stable. Should these patients be returned home, perhaps with the assurance that they are not yet ready for active remediation but will be recalled at intervals to assess the optimum moment to give volume therapy? This may yield better results in terms of therapy hours expended, for both the patient and financing bodies.

During long-term follow-up it was gratifying to note continuing improvement in all those patients who had achieved the self-practice level. Most had been extremely faithful to their task, spending some part of every day in written and spoken exercises over a two-year and even three-year period. Many still expressed frustration at their inability to achieve perfection and indeed those who have suffered more serious forms of the syndrome will never attain it. That they could continue such a demanding task over such an extended period must surely indicate that communication is one of man's most basic needs.

APPENDIX A

FACILITATING PHRASES

Groups marked with an asterisk may be initially difficult.

	W
I don't know	*why*
Peace or	*war*
It's a long, long	*way*

	w . . . t
Water is	*wet*
Black and	*white*
Can't you	*wait*
A bushel of	*wheat*

	w . . . d
A log of	*wood*
Six metres	*wide*
I give you my	*word*
A thistle's a	*weed*

	w . . . p*
The jockey has a	*whip*
The wood will	*warp*
Please don't	*weep*

	w . . . b
A spider's	*web*

	w . . . k*
Strong or	*weak*
I'll go for a	*walk*
Are you	*awake*
This is hard	*work*

	w . . . g	
She wears a blonde		*wig*

---

	w . . . n	
A glass of		*wine*
I hope I		*win*
It's so cold in the		*winter*
Close the		*window*

---

	w . . . m	
The weather is		*warm*
It's only a		*whim*

---

	w . . . l	
A ball of		*wool*
Yes! I certainly		*will*
Turn the		*wheel*
A brick		*wall*

---

	w . . . s	
For better or		*worse*

---

	w . . . st	
East or		*west*
What a		*waste*

---

	w . . . sh*	
I must go and		*wash*
I'll grant you your		*wish*

---

	w . . . ch*	
Wind your		*watch*
I can't decide		*which* one to choose

---

	w . . . j*	
He earns a good		*wage*

---

	w . . . f*	
Husband and		*wife*
The ship's at the		*wharf*

52

*w . . . v**

A weaver can	*weave*
Give me a	*wave*

M

Give it to	*me*
The month of	*May*
I need some	*more*

m . . . t

Wipe your feet on the	*mat*
A butcher sells	*meat*
I think it	*might* rain
He was my best	*mate*

m . . . d

I'm in a bad	*mood*
My bed has been	*made*
I think it's	*mad*
Ancient and	*mod*ern

*m . . . p**

You need a road	*map*
The broom and the	*mop*

*m . . . k**

What did you	*make*
He made his	*mark*
Michael or	*Mike*

m . . . g

A cup or a	*mug*

m . . . n

This book is	*mine*
A boy or a	*man*
Don't be so	*mean* with your *money*

53

| | *m . . . m* | |
| Dad and | | *mum* |

	m . . . l*	
A flour		*mill*
He ran a		*mile*
I enjoyed that nice		*meal*

	m . . . s	
A cat and a		*mouse*
What a		*mess*
Hit or		*miss*

| | *m . . . sh** | |
| I won't eat that | | *mush* |

	m . . . ch*	
Strike a		*match*
Don't give me so		*much*

	P	
Rich or		*poor*
An apple		*pie*

	p . . . t	
A tea		*pot*
Give the dog a		*pat*
The whole or a		*part*
Let's have a		*party*
What a		*pity*

| | *p . . . d* | |
| The account has been | | *paid* |

	p . . . p	
A dog or a		*pup*
It went off		*pop*
An orange		*pip*

54

	p . . . k
Take your	*pick*
Roast	*pork*
I must go and	*pack*
I keep it in my	*pock*et

	p . . . g
A big, fat	*pig*

	p . . . n
A needle or a	*pin*
Are you in	*pain*
I write with a	*pen*

	p . . . l*
Swallow this	*pill*
Push and	*pull*
You look	*pale*
Orange	*peel*

	p . . . s
Either bid or	*pass*
War and	*peace*

	p . . . sh*
Pull and	*push*

	p . . . ch*
It's as black as	*pitch*
My pants need a	*patch*
The front	*porch*
Apricot or	*peach*

	p . . . j*
Turn over the	*page*

	p . . . th*
A concrete	*path*

55

B

I was stung by a	*bee*
He is a	*bore*
What did you	*buy*
He never said	*boo*

b . . . t

A cricket	*bat*
That dog will	*bite*
A rowing	*boat*
Just a little	*bit*
This lemon is	*bitt*er
Bread and	*butt*er

b . . . d

Good or	*bad*
Go to	*bed*
What will you	*bid*
A rose	*bud*

b . . . b

A baby's	*bib*
Robert or	*Bob*

b . . . k

Read a good	*book*
Ride a motor	*bike*
That dog will	*bark*
The bird has a sharp	*beak*

b . . . k

Front or	*back*
Bread from the	*bak*er

b . . . g

Small or	*big*
A paper	*bag*
Sit up and	*beg*
I saw an old	*begg*ar

	b . . . n
Where were you	born
A rubbish	bin
Where have you	been

	b . . . nd
A brass	band
Her legs are	bandy

	b . . . l*
Catch the	ball
Ring the	bell
Pay the	bill
A cow or a	bull

| | *b . . . s* |
| I'll go by | bus |

| | *b . . . st* |
| I like this one the | best |

| | *b . . . sh** |
| Way out in the | bush (Australian idiom) |

	b . . . ch
A dog or a	bitch
Meat from the	butcher

| | *b . . . j* |
| He is wearing his | badge |

	b . . . th*
A shower or a	bath
I'll have	both
I won't	bother

	T
One	two
A collar and	tie

57

t . . . t

My shoes are too   *tight*
A jam   *tart*

t . . . d

Edward or   *Ted*
The knot is   *tied*

t . . . p*

Bottom or   *top*
I'll give you a   *tip*

t . . . t

Turn on the   *tap*
A typist can   *type*

t . . . b

Grow the tree in a   *tub*

t . . . k*

A cross or a   *tick*
A nail or a   *tack*
Give or   *take*
I'll teach you to   *talk*

t . . . g*

It needs a sharp   *tug*
A lion or a   *tiger*

t . . . n

Six, seven, eight, nine   *ten*
It must weigh a   *ton*
A box or a   *tin*
I'll get a sun   *tan*

t . . . m

Tell me the   *time*
A cricket   *team*
Thomas or   *Tom*
Wild or   *tame*

58

	t . . . l *
Ten feet	*tall*
I won't	*tell*
Put the change in the	*till*
A hammer is a	*tool*
The dog wagged his	*tail*

	t . . . s
Don't argue the	*toss*

	t . . . st
Did you pass the	*test*
Does it have a nice	*taste*

	t . . . ch
He lit up his	*torch*
I'm right out of	*touch*
I'll learn if you	*teach*
He's a very good	*teach*er

	t . . . f *
This meat is too	*tough*

	t . . . th *
I must clean my	*teeth*

	D
What can I	*do*
It's a very warm	*day*
Open the	*door*

	d . . . t
What is the	*date*
You must pay your	*debt*
It was never in	*doubt*

	d . . . d
Mum and	*dad*
Alive or	*dead*
Yes! I	*did*

	d . . . p	
A lucky		*dip*

	d . . . k	
Light or		*dark*
A sitting		*duck*
The ship's in		*dock*

	d . . . g	
Get a spade and		*dig*

	d . . . n	
My work is		*done*
A fox has a		*den*
What a loud		*din*
I must eat my		*dinner*

	d . . . m	
Bright or		*dim*
Deaf and		*dumb*

	d . . . l*	
The weather is		*dull*

	d . . . z	
Yes! It		*does*

	d . . . sh	
A very tasty		*dish*
I must		*dash*

	d . . . ch	
Hans is		*Dutch*
Dig a deep		*ditch*

	d . . . v*	
He did a high		*dive*
As gentle as a		*dove*
Dad and		*Dave* (Australian idiom)

60

L

High and	*low*
Obey the	*law*
The hens won't	*lay*

l . . . t

Switch on the	*light*
Early or	*late*
A house to	*let*
Write me a	*let*ter
I'll·see you	*lat*er

l . . . d

As heavy as	*lead*
He's a good	*lad*
Climb up the	*ladder*
Take the	*lead*
Follow the	*leader*

l . . . p

My top	*lip*
The cat's on my	*lap*

l . . . b

Liberal or	*Lab*or (Australian idiom)

l . . . k

Take a good	*look*
They both look	a*like*
We swam in the	*lake*
That tap will	*leak*

l . . . g

He broke his left	*leg*
Jump over the	*log*

l . . . n

Rule a straight	*line*
Fat or	*lean*
He arranged a bank	*loan*

	l . . . m	
That horse is	*lame*	
Oranges and	*lemons*	
As quiet as a	*lamb*	

	l . . . s	
Profit and	*loss*	
More or	*less*	

| | *l . . . st* | |
| First or | *last* | |

	l . . . ch	
Lift up the	*latch*	
Left in the	*lurch*	

	l . . . f*	
Not on your	*life* (Australian idiom)	
We had a good	*laugh*	

	l . . . v*	
Where does he	*live*	
Hate or	*love*	

	K/C	
Drive the	*car*	
The car	*key*	
An apple	*core*	

	c/k . . . t*	
A pussy	*cat*	
A knife will	*cut*	
A rain	*coat*	
Go fly a	*kite*	

	c/k . . . d	
A cow chews its	*cud*	
I wish I	*could*	
A goat and a	*kid*	
Play your best	*card*	

62

	c/k . . . p
A saucer and	*cup*
A hat or a	*cap*
Brass or	*copp*er

	c/k . . . b
A taxi	*cab*
A wolf and a	*cub*

	c/k . . . k*
A birthday	*cake*
That donkey will	*kick*
She's a good	*cook*

	c/k . . . n
Beer comes in a	*can*
Kith and	*kin*
I feel very	*keen*
A cob of	*corn*

	c/k . . . m
Go or	*come*
The sea is	*calm*

	c/k . . . l*
A telephone	*call*
Guns can	*kill*
Warm or	*cool*

	c/k . . . s
Give Grandpa a	*kiss*
Swear and	*curse*
A race	*course* (Australian)

| | *c . . . st* |
| What does it | *cost* |

| | *c . . . sh* |
| Will you pay | *cash* |

	c . . . ch	
You throw and I'll		*catch*

	c . . . f*	
That's a nasty		*cough*
A cow and a		*calf*

	c . . . v	
Get a knife and I'll		*carve*
He hid in a		*cave*
Go slowly on the		*curve*

	G	
Stop and		*go*
Happy and		*gay*

	g . . . t	
Shut the		*gate*
What have you		*got*
A billy		*goat*

	g . . . d	
Bad or		*good*

	g . . . p	
Close up the		*gap*

	g . . . n	
I'll shoot with this		*gun*
He's been here and		*gone*
Do it		a*gain*

	g . . . m	
Play the		*game*
Chewing		*gum*

	g . . . l*	
He scored a		*goal*
A boy and a		*girl*
That bird's a sea		*gull*

	g . . . s
Turn off the	*gas*

	g . . . st
Be polite to your	*guest*
I saw a	*ghost*

	g . . . v
Some take but some	*give*

	N
Yes or	*no*
Far or	*near*

	n . . . t
Day and	*night*
Tie the	*knot*
Get wool and	*knit*
A bolt and a	*nut*
Tidy and	*neat*

	n . . . d
I'll give you the	*nod* (Australian idiom)
What do we	*need*

	n . . . p
I'll have a short	*nap*
The dog took a	*nip*

	n . . . k
He has a stiff	*neck*
It took a bad	*knock* (Australian idiom)

	n . . . g
Don't	*nag*

	n . . . n
Six, seven, eight	*nine*
I have	*none*

	n . . . m	
What is your		*name*
My foot has gone		*numb*

	n . . . l	
The score is		*nil*
The River		*Nile*
A hammer and		*nail*

| | *n . . . s* | |
| That isn't | | *nice* |

	n . . . st	
Birds in the		*nest*
It tastes rather		*nasty*

| | *n . . . s(z)* | |
| Blow your | | *nose* |

	n . . . f	
Set a fork and a		*knife*
I've had		*enough*

	S	
Can you		*see*
That isn't		*so*
My leg is		*sore*
What did you		*say*

	s . . . t	
Sit on the		*seat*
I've got good eye-		*sight*
She's a good		*sort* (Australian idiom)
Friday and		*Saturday*

	s . . . d	
Isn't it		*sad*
I heard what you		*said*
All of a		*sudden*
She sighed and she		*sighed*

	s . . . p
A cake of	*soap*
A bowl of	*soup*
A warm drink for	*supp*er

	s . . . k
Do you feel	*sick*
My shoe and my	*sock*
He got the	*sack* (Australian idiom)

	s . . . g
That mattress will	*sag*

	s . . . n
It's a wicked, wicked	*sin*
Is he quite	*sane*
Take a pen and	*sign*

	s . . . nd
They sunbaked on the	*sand*
Did you hear that loud	*sound*

	s . . . m
Are they all the	*same*
This is a hard	*sum*
It's hot in the	*summ*er
Just leave it to	*simm*er

	*s . . . l**
We will go for a	*sail*
Put it on the window	*sill*
Don't be so	*sill*y

	*s . . . f**
I don't think that is	*safe*
They swam in the	*surf*

	*s . . . v**
How much money did you	*save*

67

SH

My sock and my   *shoe*
Row for the   *shore*
The baby is   *shy*
Let us go to a   *show*

sh . . . t

Get a gun and   *shoot*
Open and   *shut*
Change the   *sheet*

sh . . . d

The sun or the   *shade*
A garden   *shed*
Yes! You   *should*

sh . . . p

This knife is   *sharp*
He's in good   *shape* (Australian idiom)
A boat or a   *ship*

sh . . . b

My clothes are so   *shabby*

sh . . . k

It gave me a   *shock*
Look out for the   *shark*

sh . . . g

A spoonful of   *sugar*

sh . . . n

The sun will   *shine*

sh . . . m

What a   *shame*

sh . . . l

Yes! I   *shall*
A sea   *shell*

68

	*sh . . . s/(**s**)*
Socks and	*shoes*

	sh . . . v
I'll have a shower and a	*shave*

	CH
Sit on the	*chair*

	ch . . . t
It's wrong to	*cheat*
Can you read the	*chart*
Let's have a	*chat*

	ch . . . p
Expensive or	*cheap*

	ch . . . k
What a	*cheek* (idiomatic)
Pay by	*cheque* (**check**)

	ch . . . n
A double	*chin*
A link in the	*chain*

	ch . . . m
She's full of	*charm*

	ch . . . l*
Don't catch a	*chill*

	ch . . . s
Run and I'll give	*chase*
A game of	*chess*
Make your	*choice*

	ch . . . st
A cold in the	*chest*

| | *ch . . . ch* |
| Pray in the | *church* |

| | *ch . . . j* |
| Who is in | *charge* |

	J
Joseph or	*Joe*
Jump for	*joy*
A glass	*jar*

| | *j . . . t* |
| We flew there by | *jet* |

| | *j . . . b* |
| He has a good | *job* |

	j . . . k
I'll tell you a	*joke*
His name is	*Jack*

| | *j . . . g* |
| The milk is in the | *jug* |

	j . . . n
A bottle of	*gin*
They called her	*Jane*
Is it Jack or	*John*

	j . . . m
James or	*Jim*
Strawberry	*jam*

	j . . . mp
Run and	*jump*
Put on your	*jump*er (idiom)

	j . . . l*
The prisoner is in	*jail*
Jack and	*Jill*
A diamond is a	*jewel*

70

| | *j . . . j* |
| You be the | *judge* |

	R
The lions will	*roar*
All standing in a	*row*
Is it wheat or	*rye*

	r . . . t
Left or	*right*
A mouse or a	*rat*
What a lot of	*rot*

	r . . . d
Get a book and	*read*
Drive on the	*road*
Is it pink or	*red*
Don't be so	*rude*

	r . . . p
This apple is	*ripe*
A skipping	*rope*

	r . . . b
Give it a good	*rub*
A pencil and	*rubb*er
A robber will	*rob*
That bird is a	*rob*in

	r . . . k
A hoe and a	*rake*
Put it up on the	*rack*
That car is a	*wreck*

	r . . . g
A carpet or	*rug*
A piece of old	*rag*

71

	r . . . n
It is going to	*rain*
Walk—don't	*run*
I ran and I	*ran*

	r . . . m
A bottle of	*rum*
The Pope lives in	*Rome*
A sheep and a	*ram*
Come into the	*room*
Don't listen to	*rum*our

	r . . . l *
A train on the	*rail*s
Follow the	*rule*s
Keep it straight with a	*rule*r
I'll have a bread	*roll*

	r . . . s (**s**)
A bowl of	*rice*

	r . . . z
A red, red,	*rose*

	r . . . st
I'll have a nice	*rest*
That tin will	*rust*

	r . . . sh
Measles is a	*rash*
Please don't	*rush*

	r . . . ch
Poor or	*rich*
It is out of	*reach*

	r . . .f *
A leak in the	*roof*
Smooth or	*rough*

	F
One, two, three	*four*

	f . . . t
It measures a	*foot*
He's a victim of	*fate*
Thin or	*fat*
Please don't	*fight*

	f . . . d
It's only a	*fad*
Enjoy your	*food*
That colour will	*fade*
That car is a	*Ford*

	f . . . n
The weather is	*fine*
An electric	*fan*
This isn't much	*fun*
I think it's	*funny*

	f . . . k
A knife and a	*fork*

	f . . . g
I'm lost in the	*fog*

	f . . . m
He lives on a	*farm*
He is a	*farmer*
Sign this	*form*

	f . . . l*
Empty or	*full*
I won't	*fail*
Mind you don't	*fall*

73

f . . . s

Wash your	*face*
Taken by	*force*
Don't make a	*fuss*
I'm not	*fussy*

f . . . st

Don't go so	*fast*
What a wonderful	*feast*

f . . . ch

Dog—go and	*fetch*

f . . . v

One, two, three, four	*five*
Do me a	*favour*

V

v . . . t

I'll cast my	*vote*
Take the dog to the	*vet*

v . . . n

It's all in	*vain*
A truck or a	*van*
The grape is a	*vine*

v . . . l

A bridal	*veil*
Beef or	*veal*
It is very good	*value*

v . . . s (**z**)

Put the flowers in the	*vase*

v . . . s (**s**)

I've almost lost my	*voice*

Gradual Introduction of Blends in Rhyming Sheets

*p*each	*b*each	*t*each	reach	*pr*each		
*h*ill	*m*ill	*p*ill	*w*ill	*k*ill	s*t*ill	s*k*ill
*h*ail	mail	*p*ale	*w*ail	sale	s*t*ale	s*c*ale
*h*all	*c*all	tall	*w*all	*f*all	s*t*all	s*m*all
*h*old	*c*old	told	*m*ould	*f*old	sold	s*c*old
*h*and	*b*and	*l*and	*s*and	s*t*and	*gr*and	*br*and
*b*ust	*d*ust	*m*ust	*r*ust	*tr*ust	*cr*ust	*thr*ust
*d*amp	*c*amp	*l*amp	s*t*amp	*cr*amp	*tr*amp	
rock	*l*ock	*kn*ock	*sh*ock	s*t*ock	*cr*ock	*cl*ock
*th*ick	*l*ick	*pr*ick	*br*ick	*tr*ick	*cl*ick	s*t*ick
*f*etch	wretch	s*k*etch	s*tr*etch			
*t*ight	*l*ight	*f*ight	*fl*ight	*fr*ight	*pl*ight	*bl*ight	*br*ight
*h*umble	*t*umble	*r*umble	*f*umble	s*t*umble	*gr*umble	*cr*umble

Changing the Terminal

wi*de*	wi*ne*	wi*pe*	wi*se*	whi*te*	whi*le*
ri*de*	ri*ce*	ri*pe*	ri*se*	ri*ght*	
fi*ne*	fi*ve*	fi*re*	fi*le*	fi*ght*	
ca*ne*	ca*ve*	ca*me*	ca*se*		
grow	grow*n*	grow*er*	grow*th*	grow*ing*	
post	post*s*	post*er*	post*ed*	post*ing*	
burn	burn*s*	burn*er*	burn*ed*	burn*ing*	

Double Syllable with Stable Prefix—Stable Suffix

be*come*	be*long*	be*ware*	be*side*	be*fore*	
re*pair*	re*move*	re*mind*	re*tire*	re*fuse*	re*quest*
dis*like*	dis*miss*	dis*may*	dis*grace*	dis*cover*	
per*haps*	per*son*	per*form*	per*fume*	per*fect*	

Note: As the patient becomes more comfortable with the double syllable he no longer needs the support of a strong ideational content

*pi*llow	*ho*llow	*fo*llow	*fe*llow	*ye*llow	*swa*llow
*com*ic	*pan*ic	*traff*ic	*pub*lic	*pic*nic	
*fur*nish	*fi*nish	*pu*nish	*po*lish	*var*nish	*Span*ish
*in*side	*out*side	*up*side	*be*side		
*use*less	*care*less	*name*less	*shame*less		
*aw*ful	*care*ful	*plenti*ful	*beauti*ful		

Working Towards the Polysyllabic

re*ward*	re*mind*	re*late*	re*lation*	re*member*	re*membering*
con*tent*	con*tain*	con*tainer*	con*tinue*	con*sider*	con*sideration*
com*plain*	com*plaining*	com*plete*	com*pletion*		
im*pact*	im*agine*	im*agination*	im*possible*	im*itate*	im*itation*
inter*view*	inter*rupt*	inter*ruption*	inter*fere*	inter*ference*	

Suggested Compound Words with Strong Ideational Value

home	*sick*	—	homesick
sun	*light*	—	sunlight
arm	*chair*	—	armchair
pan	*cake*	—	pancake
rose	*bud*	—	rosebud
cow	*boy*	—	cowboy
house	*wife*	—	housewife
free	*way*	—	freeway
water	*fall*	—	waterfall
book	*case*	—	bookcase
sun	*shine*	—	sunshine
sun	*day*	—	Sunday
foot	*ball*	—	football
tea	*spoon*	—	teaspoon
rail	*way*	—	railway
rain	*bow*	—	rainbow
friend	*ship*	—	friendship
bed	*room*	—	bedroom
watch	*man*	—	watchman
life	*saver*	—	lifesaver
after	*noon*	—	afternoon
pad	*lock*	—	padlock
butter	*fly*	—	butterfly
some	*thing*	—	something
any	*thing*	—	anything
under	*stand*	—	understand
mouse	*trap*	—	mousetrap

APPENDIX B

GRADED POLYSYLLABIC WORDS ILLUSTRATING PHONETIC ASSISTANCE

Dotted lines indicate the patient should continue to voice the last syllable until the oral position is found for the following one. Articulatory position is mastered first through a wider range of movement, ie **shun**, then refined to a narrower range, ie **shn**.

tim . . . id	**more . . . bid**	**liv . . . id**	**ridge . . . id**
timid	*morbid*	*livid*	*rigid*

fridge . . . id
frigid

me . . . zhu	**le . . . zhu**	**tre . . . zhu**
measure	*leisure*	*treasure*

nay . . . chu	**pick . . . chu**	**cull . . . chu**	**ad . . . ven . . . chu**
nature	*picture*	*culture*	*adventure*

man . . . shun	**dick . . . shun**	**fick . . . shun**
mansion	*diction*	*fiction*

am . . . bi . . . shun	**low . . . kay . . . shun**
ambition	*location*

con . . . few . . . shun	**re . . . sep . . . shun**
confusion	*reception*

dick . . . tay . . . shun	**pro . . . duck . . . shun**
dictation	*production*

in . . . for . . . may . . . shun
information

core . . . shus	**vi . . . shus**	**spay . . . shus**
cautious	*vicious*	*spacious*

con . . . shus	**pre . . . shus**	**un . . . con . . . shus**
conscious	*precious*	*unconscious*

dee . . . li . . . shus	**sus . . . pi . . . shus**	**in . . . feck . . . shus**
delicious	*suspicious*	*infectious*

mar . . . ve . . . luss	**rid . . . ick . . . you . . . luss**
marvellous	*ridiculous*

77

poor . . . russ
porous

boy . . . stir . . . russ
boisterous

ad . . . vent . . . you . . . russ
adventurous

con . . . tin . . . you . . . us
continuous

dee . . . sid . . . you . . . us
deciduous

stren . . . you . . . us
strenuous

bill . . . yus
bilious

con . . . tay . . . jus
contagious

so . . . shall
social

off . . . i . . . shall
official

super . . . fi . . . shall
superficial

ee . . . sen . . . shall
essential

con . . . shense
conscience

pay . . . shense
patience

im . . . pay . . . shense
impatience

APPENDIX C

ORAL POSITIONS

Lips

m

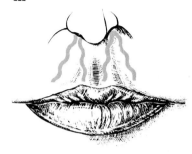

Teeth + Breath

s **z**

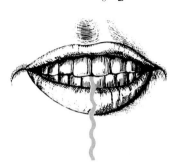

p **b**

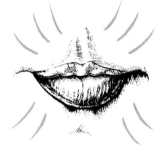

Tongue

t **d**

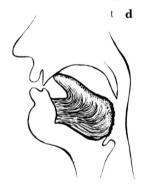

w

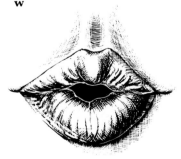

k **g**

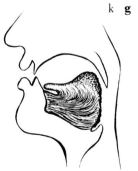

ORAL POSITIONS

Tongue
n

Lips + Teeth + Breath
ch **j**

r

v

Lips + Teeth + Breath
sh

Tongue + Breath
th

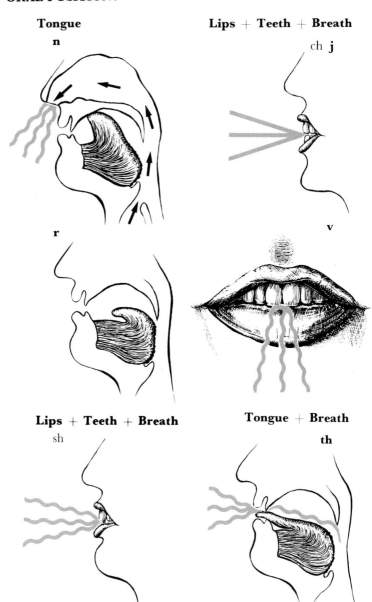

DATE DUE